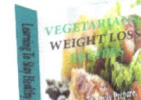

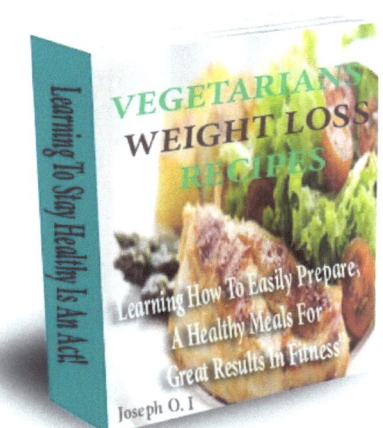

Terms and Conditions

LEGAL NOTICE

The Publisher has strived to be as accurate and complete as possible in the creation of this report, notwithstanding the fact that he does not warrant or represent at any time that the contents within are accurate due to the rapidly changing nature of the Internet.

While all attempts have been made to verify information provided in this publication, the Publisher assumes no responsibility for errors, omissions, or contrary interpretation of the subject matter herein. Any perceived slights of specific persons, peoples, or organizations are unintentional.

In practical advice books, like anything else in life, there are no guarantees of income made. Readers are cautioned to reply on their own judgment about their individual circumstances to act accordingly.

This book is not intended for use as a source of legal, business, accounting or financial advice. All readers are advised to seek services of competent professionals in legal, business, accounting and finance fields.

You are encouraged to print this book for easy reading.

Table Of Contents

Foreword

Chapter 1:
Healthy Meal Basics

Chapter 2:
How Black Beans Help And A Black Bean Recipe

Chapter 3:
How Oats Help And A Oat Recipe

Chapter 4:
How Avocados Help And A Avocado Recipe

Chapter 5:
How Salmon Helps And A Salmon Recipe

Chapter 6:
How Eating The Right Foods Helps Those Pounds Melt Away

Wrapping Up

Foreword

The perception that thin people are healthy people could not be further from the truth; though in contrast fat people are really mostly unhealthy people are quite true. Therefore in order to be healthy and stay healthy one should really concentrate on the nutritional value of the foods being consumed rather than the amounts. Better your health here.

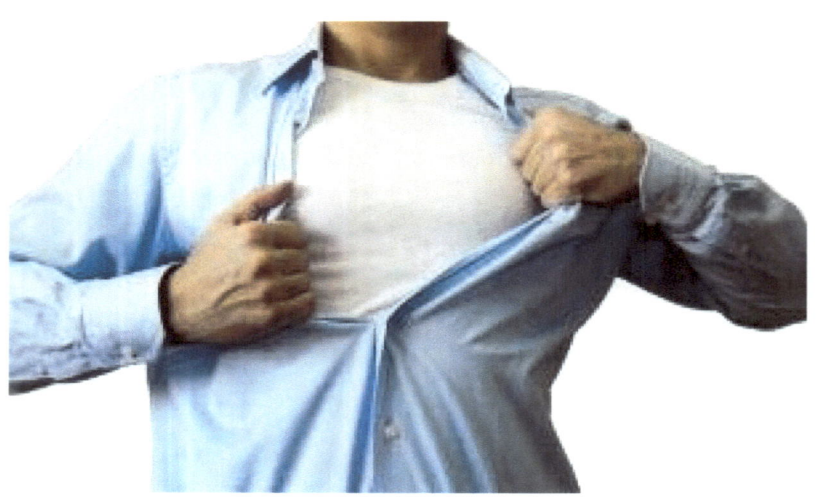

Vegetarians Weight Loss Recipes

Learning How To Easily Prepare, A Healthy Meals For Great Results In Fitness

Chapter 1:

Healthy Meal Basics

Synopsis

Ideally small amount of food intake is best but only if these amounts consists of nutritionally balanced and healthy elements.

Exploring the various nutritional basics of each category within the food groups helps the individual to make informed choices regarding the food consumed. Upon gaining this understanding the next step would be to make the changes needed but doing so gradually would better reap positive results as opposed to drastically making the change which the body may accept for a short period of time and then reject in the long run.

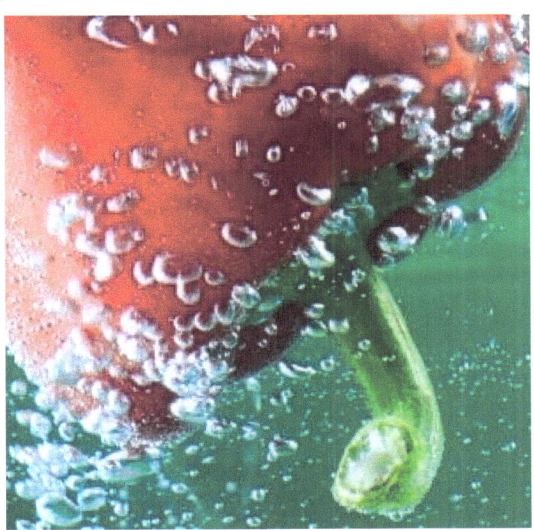

The Basics

Finding the foods in simpler and more variety and freshness though still maintaining some of the favorite ingredients helps the body accept the new food intake with less of a shock to the system both body and mind.

Making these changes over a period of time is also necessary if the effort is to remain continuous. Substituting certain unhealthy ingredients with healthier one while still maintain the general recipe is also recommended.

Totally avoiding unhealthy foods is of course ideal but really quite an unrealistic pressure as it causes the individual to feel deprived and stressed, therefore a better alternative would be to wean themselves slowly off the item instead.

Learning to eat in smaller portions also helps the individual start the journey towards healthy eating. For some cutting out certain foods may be such a difficult effort that the next best solution would be to try and cut down the portions. Also developing the habit of avoiding heavier meals towards the end of a day is also wise.

Chapter 2:

How Black Beans Help And A Black Bean Recipe

Synopsis

As more and more people become aware of this particular food called the black bean the interest in it has also become heightened. Originating from Mexico and very much a part of the South American diet, these black beans have been proven to be quite a nutritionally pack food group indeed. Today it is popularly found in most restaurants and homes in various forms such as salads, staples and other delicious dishes.

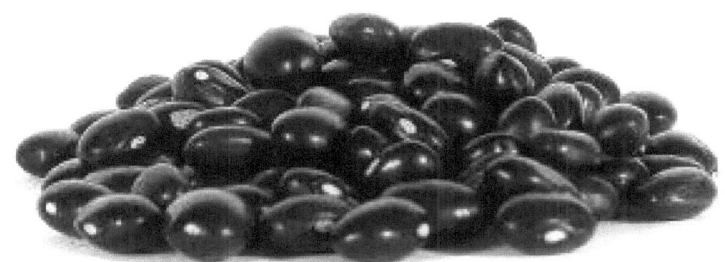

Black Beans

The black beans consists of high protein and fiber contents and is considered very nourishing as both these essential elements are present within one food item. Fiber and proteins are considered very important to the wholesome function of a healthy body. Besides this it also has flavonoid anti oxidants content which assist the body avoid oxygen related damage. Black beans also consists of omega 3 fatty acids and has a high nutritional value.

Black beans are also very easy to incorporate into most meals as it has a basic flavor of rich smokiness, which gives added character to any dish. The velvet texture, shape and color hold well during cooking and makes for a very interesting looking ingredient indeed.

Black Bean Salad

Ingredients
The Salad - (I try to keep the cuts not too much bigger than the beans & corn - for appearance & to get a little of everything in a spoonful)
2 lbs. black beans (I have a pressure cooker, but go ahead, use 2 15 oz. cans, well-rinsed.)

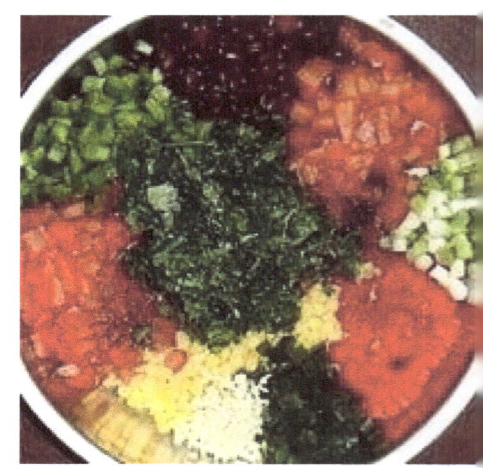

2 lbs. cooked sweet corn, cut from the cob (OK, you can use 2 - 15 oz. cans of whole kernel corn or 2 lbs. of frozen corn, drained)

8 green onions, diced

2 cloves garlic, large, minced

2-3 jalapeno peppers, cleaned, diced (more if you like)

1 green Bell pepper, cleaned, diced (I also sometimes add a small sweet red pepper, for both sweetness & color)

1 ripe avocado, large, pitted, peeled and diced

1 jar (4 oz) pimentos, drained

3 tomatoes, seeded & diced

1C fresh cilantro, chopped

Sea salt & fresh cracked black pepper to taste The Dressing

3 T fresh lime juice

2 T fresh orange juice

2-1/2 tsp lime zest 1/2 tsp ground cumin

Sea salt & fresh cracked black pepper to taste

Directions

Combine all the salad ingredients in a large bowl. Season with the salt & pepper. Whisk the dressing vigorously to incorporate. Add the dressing to the salad and gently toss to combine everything. Chill until ready to serve. Lightly toss again prior to serving.

Prepare this salad at least 4 hours prior to serving to let everything - except the avocado - marry joyfully in the bowl.

You do want to let the avocado bathe in the lime juice of the dressing - better presentation that way, and you can store the avocado pieces in a small container. Then, pour the dressing off the avocado and mix the salad with the dressing, then dress the top of the salad with the avocado pieces at service.

Very pretty dish & the absence of any oil seems to make all the veggies sparkle in a light citrus glow. You want this salad well chilled, but if you don't bathe the avocados in the dressing first, they will end up looking like grey lumps of pork as the air hits them.

Chapter 3:

How Oats Help And A Oat Recipe

Synopsis

Eating oats to enhance good health is not something new but has been practice through time. Oats is a very simple ingredient with far reaching positive effects and benefits.

Oats within a diet plan provides a wide range of important health benefits which cannot be duplicated by any other food item singularly. Being a significant dietary fiber source, oats consists of soluble and half soluble fibers which help to keep blood cholesterol levels effectively under control.

Some of the areas where oats has been known to be beneficial are in improving heart conditions, regulating blood sugar levels, functioning as anti cancer fighters, keeping blood pressure under control, maintaining regular and healthy bowel functions, helping in weight control, boosting athletic performances, and in general health and longevity.

Oats

Oats is also a food item that is rather hardy and can be grown in poor soil conditions which is of course another plus in terms of its availability. The various processes that the oat has to be subjected to before it reaches the dining table does not cause its nutritional value to decrease rather it is able to maintain its concentrated high fiber and nutrient base.

Oats can be a great day starter in the form of a piping bowl of oatmeal which can be more flavorful with the addition of fresh fruits, nuts or the dried fruits variety. It can also be used to make oat meal cookies which are usually a huge hit with kids and adults alike. Breads and muffins can also have the addition of healthy oats to it as with poultry stuffing too.

Golden Honey Oat Bread Recipe

Ingredients
1 1/4 cups and 2 tablespoons water, room temperature (70 to 90°F.)
 1/2 cup rolled oats or barley
flakes 1/4 cup flax seed cracked
2 cups unbleached flour
3/4 cup whole wheat flour
2 tablespoons vital wheat gluten
1 tablespoon powdered milk

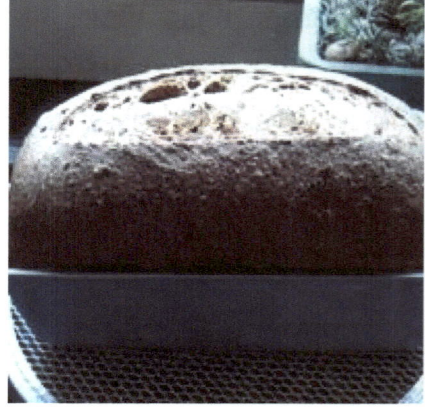

2 tablespoons honey

1 1/8 teaspoon instant yeast

2 1/2 tablespoons canola oil

2 teaspoons salt

Directions

Equipment: A 9 by 5 inch/ 7 cup bread pan, coated lightly with cooking spray. A baking stone set toward the bottom rung and a cast-iron pan on the floor of the oven.

Step 1: Make the dough (Bread Machine)

In the bread machine container, combine water, oats, and cracked flax and mix to moisten. Then let sit covered for a minimum of 15 minutes.

In a medium bowl, whisk together the flours, gluten, powdered milk, and yeast.

Add the honey, and oil to the oat mixture and then the flour mixture. Mix 3 minutes and allow to rest for 20. If your bread machine always restarts with a 3 minute mix allow it to do so while adding the salt and then go into the kneading cycle for 4 minutes. If it starts with the kneading cycle also run it for 4 minutes, adding the salt at the beginning of the kneading cycle.

Step 2: Let the dough rise

Using an oiled spatula or dough scraper, scrape the dough into a 2 quart container with cover or bowl, greased lightly with cooking spray or oil. Push down the dough and lightly spray or oil the top of the dough. It will be 4 cups /943 grams/33 ounces.). Cover the container with a lid or plastic wrap. With a piece of tape, mark where double the height would be. Allow the dough to rise (ideally at 80 to 82°F/28°C) until doubled, about 1 hour, 15 min. For extra strength and elasticity, you can stretch it after the first 30 minutes. To achieve a moist and warm temperature I put a small container of very hot water—about 1 cup--under a plastic box to create a proofer and change the water every 20 to 30 minutes. (You can retard the dough overnight after the first rise by gently deflating it and refrigerating it but it seems to rise best when baked the same day. If you refrigerate it overnight, remove it to room temperature. For about an hour before shaping.

Step 3: Shape the dough and let it rise
Turn the dough onto a lightly floured counter and press it down to flatten it slightly. It will still be sticky but use only as much flour as absolutely necessary. Shape it into a log and allow it to relax covered for 20 minutes. (This is essential for an evenly shaped dough.)

Shape the dough into a loaf set it into the prepared baking pan. It will be about 3/4 inches from the top of the pan.

Cover the shaped dough with the plastic box or oiled plastic wrap and allow it to rise until almost doubled and when pressed gently with a finger the depression very slowly fills in. The highest point will be about 1 1/2 inches higher than the sides of the pan. Using the plastic box and hot water it takes 1 hour 15 minutes to 1 1/2 hours. At a cooler temperature it will take longer. Meantime preheat the oven for a minimum of 40 minutes.

Step 4: Slash and bake the bread

If you like the look of a bread with a slash down the middle, with a sharp knife or straight edged razor blade, make a 1/2 inch deep slash down the top of the dough. You can also leave it unslashed. Mist the dough with water, quickly but gently set the baking sheet on the hot stone or hot baking sheet and toss 1/2 cup of ice cubes into the pan beneath. Immediately shut the door, lower the temperature to 375°F/190°C, and bake 20 minutes. Turn the dough around, tent, and continue baking 15 to 20 minutes or until the bread is golden brown and a skewer inserted in the middle comes out clean. (An instant read thermometer inserted into the center will read about 205°F.)

Step 5: Cool the bread

Unmold the bread onto a wire rack and allow it to cool, top-side-up until barely warm.

Chapter 4:

How Avocados Help And A Avocado Recipe

Synopsis

More and more today the world is looking to avocados as the next wholesome nutritious food replacement. Originating in Mexico and Central America it can now be found in many other countries like Indonesia, Philippines, Thailand, India, china, Japan, Peru and the list goes on.

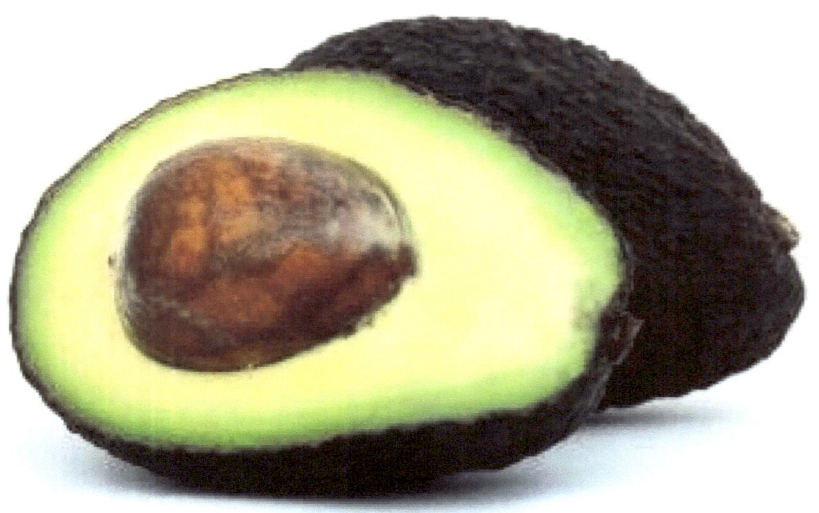

Avocado

Ranging from being able to cure certain cancer diseases to the ideal food energy source for body builders, this remarkable fruit is fast gaining the popularity it so aptly deserves.

A little known fact about the avocado is that, when the avocado fruit is mixed into salads, it aids in the absorption of all the other nutrients the salad may have in a more efficient way.

When a comparison is made with other fruits the avocado wins all the time, as the fruit that is better able to allow the nutrients to be absorbed and also for its high content of many different nutrients.

The avocado is also considered a "meaty" fruit as the creamy like texture is rich and quite adequately makes for a good meal or an accompanying ingredient that enhances and enriches any dish.

For those wanting to avoid certain foods for health or religious reasons the avocado is known to be a good substitute as it contains adequate amounts of meat proteins, fat oils, vitamins and minerals.

Avocado Dip
Ingredients

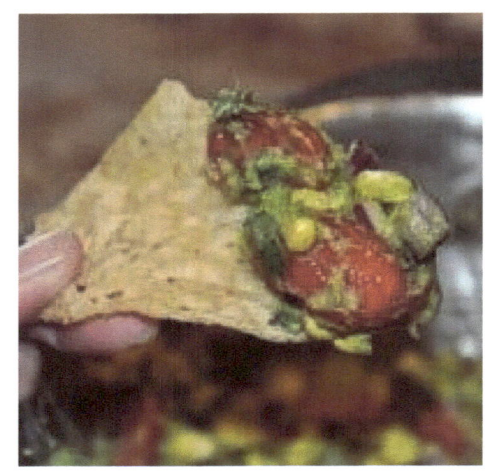

4 avocados

1 red onion

1/2 bunch of cilantro

1 ear of sweet corn

1 pint of sweet grape

tomatoes Juice of 1/2 lime

2 fresh jalapeno peppers

Directions

Remove avocado and dice in a bowl. Shuck corn and remove kernels from cob and add to avocado. Dice red onion, cilantro and jalapeno. Slice tomatoes in half. Add to mixture, season with salt and pepper. Cover with plastic wrap and store in fridge. Be sure to press plastic wrap to the surface of the dip to prevent browning. I also add the avocado seed to the bowl to help prevent browning.

Chapter 5:

How Salmon Helps And A Salmon Recipe

Synopsis

Consuming salmon in moderation has many health benefits, some yet to be fully explored but none the less accepted as one of the best and purest form of providing the fatty acid richness humans need. It is known to aid in the optimum health conditions that allows people to live longer and healthier lives.

The proteins found in salmon can easily be digested and absorbed into the body's system without causing any adverse effects that some other proteins have been known to cause.

The proteins which are found in the salmon are referred to as amino acids and are vital to the human health as these good fats or Omega 3 fatty acids provide the necessary balance for the body. Salmon also has vitamin A, B and D, minerals, iron, phosphorus and selenium within the content makeup.

Salmon

For those having heart problems, or recovering from a heart attack, the consumption of salmon is encouraged primarily because it aids in the lowering of bad cholesterol and replacing it with good cholesterol. Salmon also helps to repair heart damage and strengthen the heart muscles. Salmon also works as a natural antidepressant and help the brain work better while improving the memory capabilities of an individual. There is even some evidence of being able to positively affect the aging process. Salmon also helps to lower the blood sugar level which is especially beneficial to those suffering from diabetes. It also contributes to a more optimum metabolic rate. Healthy hair which is bright and shiny, good skin quality and bright eyes are all the positive benefits of consuming salmon.

Baked Salmon
Ingredients

Fresh salmon filets (allow about 1 per person)
1/3 cup orange juice
2 lemons
Salt
Pepper
Garlic powder
Italian seasoning

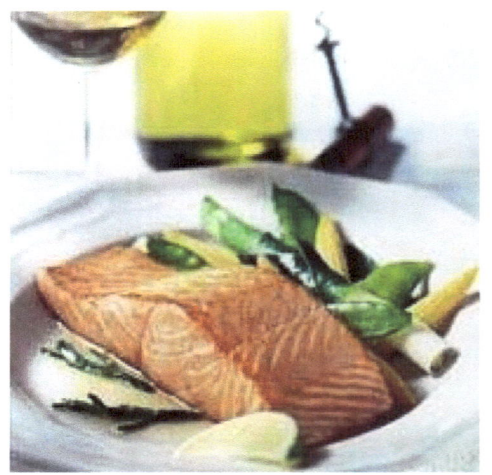

Fresh cilantro for garnishing

Directions

Preheat oven to 375 degrees

Wash & place salmon filets skin side down into deep rectangular baking dish

Mix 1/3 cup orange juice with the juice of one of the lemons; pour mixture over salmon filets in baking dish

Season each salmon filet with salt, pepper, garlic powder, and Italian seasoning to taste

Cut the second lemon in half, cut one half of lemon into slices and place slices on top of salmon filets

(The second half of this lemon will be sliced and placed on salmon after it's done)

Bake salmon filets for 15-25 minutes depending on the thickness

After baking, place filets on serving dish and place slices from the second half of the lemon on top

Garnish filets with cilantro

Chapter 6:

How Eating The Right Foods Helps Those Pounds Melt Away

Synopsis

For most people losing weight is an uphill battle and one that is often lost to tears and frustration. It is very difficult to stop eating and drinking certain things that brings pleasure to the individual, thus even trying to do so, causes stress and often failure to stick to the resolution for longer durations. Therefore exploring foods that are better and healthier would perhaps be a better alternative as compared to trying to go on a diet to lose weight.

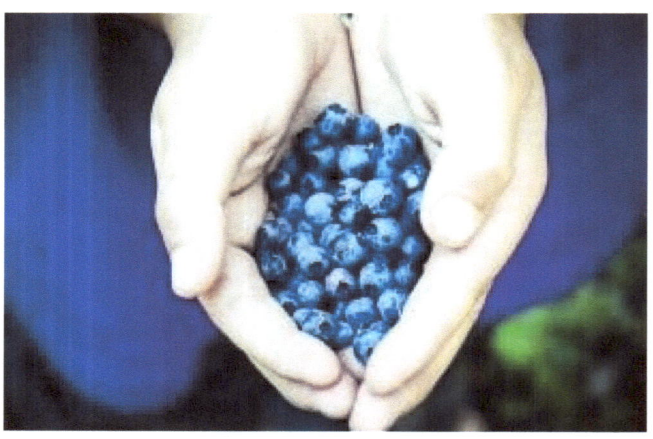

Eating Right

There are a lot of good and delicious foods that are not only good for the body but it also has the added advantage of not causing the body to retain unwanted pounds through its consumption. There are also ways preparing foods that are less likely to cause weight retention and this too should be explored if the individual is unwilling to give up eating a certain food or ingredient.

Simple measures can be taken without causing too much of a shock to the body system in the initial stages. These adjustments can then be increased as and when the body is ready and able to accept more deprivation.

Drinking a lot of water and cutting out as much sweetened food items as possible is one of the first and simplest steps to take in the quest to keep the pounds off. Keeping a food diary may also help the individual to be more aware of the foods consumed, thus creating the opportunity for the individual to make the healthier choice whenever possible. Enlisting the help of professional, such as doctors, health experts, dietitians, nutritionist can also help the individual better understand and accepts the negatives and positives of the current foods being consumed and then tailor make an appropriate diet plan with healthy food contents to encourage satisfaction without the added pounds.

Wrapping Up

Eating right helps better your health as well as help you slim down if you are trying to do that. This book has given you a good start on developing some healthy eating habits as well as some yummy recipes to get started with.

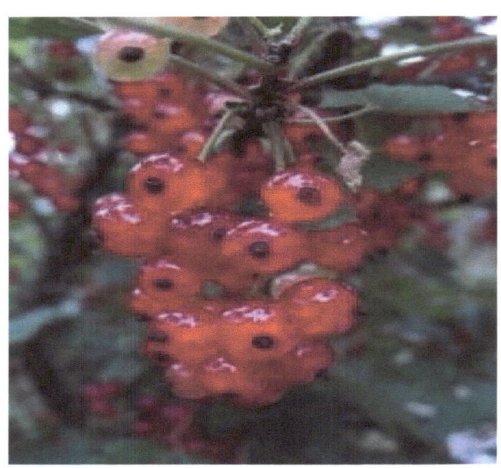

About The Author:

Name: **Mr. Joseph O Iredia,**
Contents writer, Blogger, Affiliate Marketer and Web designer.

Website Address:
www.letmoneypay.com
Email:
info@letmoneypay.com